MY DAILY FOOD DIARY

AN 8-WEEK JOURNAL FOR KIDS AGES 3–10 TO SET GOALS, TRACK MEALS, EARN REWARDS, & BUILD HEALTHY HABITS

MY DAILY FOOD DIARY
PUBLISHED BY OLIVE TREE PRESS, 2025

OLIVE TREE PRESS
HOUSTON, TEXAS
WWW.OLIVETREEPRESSCO.COM

ISBN: 978-1-965289-14-3

THIS BOOK BELONGS TO

____

WEEK 1

WEEK 1 FOOD GOALS

WEEK OF: ______________________

THIS WEEK'S GOALS

-
-
-

THIS WEEK'S REWARD FOR MEETING MY GOALS

DAILY GOAL TRACKER

(PLACE A STICKER OR CHECKMARK IF GOALS WERE ACHIEVED)

Mon Tue Wed Thu

Fri Sat Sun

DAILY FOOD DIARY

DATE: ______________________ (S) (M) (T) (W) (T) (F) (S)

TODAY'S GOALS *(IF ANY)*

GOAL MET?

BREAKFAST

LUNCH

DINNER

TOMORROW I LOOK FORWARD TO:

WATER / MILK INTAKE

TODAY I FELT...

DAILY FOOD DIARY

DATE: ______________________ (S) (M) (T) (W) (T) (F) (S)

TODAY'S GOALS *(IF ANY)*

GOAL MET?

BREAKFAST

LUNCH

DINNER

TOMORROW I LOOK FORWARD TO:

WATER / MILK INTAKE

TODAY I FELT...

DAILY FOOD DIARY

DATE: ______________________ S M T W T F S

TODAY'S GOALS *(IF ANY)*

GOAL MET?

BREAKFAST

LUNCH

DINNER

TOMORROW I LOOK FORWARD TO:

WATER / MILK INTAKE

TODAY I FELT...

DAILY FOOD DIARY

DATE: ______________________ Ⓢ Ⓜ Ⓣ Ⓦ Ⓣ Ⓕ Ⓢ

TODAY'S GOALS *(IF ANY)*

GOAL MET?

BREAKFAST

LUNCH

DINNER

TOMORROW I LOOK FORWARD TO:

WATER / MILK INTAKE

TODAY I FELT...

DAILY FOOD DIARY

DATE: ____________________ Ⓢ Ⓜ Ⓣ Ⓦ Ⓣ Ⓕ Ⓢ

TODAY'S GOALS *(IF ANY)*

GOAL MET?

BREAKFAST

LUNCH

DINNER

TOMORROW I LOOK FORWARD TO:

WATER / MILK INTAKE

TODAY I FELT...

DAILY FOOD DIARY

DATE: ______________________ S M T W T F S

TODAY'S GOALS *(IF ANY)* GOAL MET?

BREAKFAST

LUNCH

DINNER

TOMORROW I LOOK FORWARD TO:

WATER / MILK INTAKE

TODAY I FELT...

DAILY FOOD DIARY

DATE: ______________________ S M T W T F S

TODAY'S GOALS *(IF ANY)* GOAL MET?

BREAKFAST

LUNCH

DINNER

TOMORROW I LOOK FORWARD TO:

WATER / MILK INTAKE

TODAY I FELT...

WEEK 1 REFLECTION

DATE: ______________________

THIS WEEK I FELT...

NEW FOODS I TRIED THIS WEEK:

FAVORITE FOODS

LEAST FAVORITE FOODS

NEXT WEEK I LOOK FORWARD TO:

WEEK 2

WEEK 2 FOOD GOALS

WEEK OF: ______________________

THIS WEEK'S GOALS

-
-
-

THIS WEEK'S REWARD FOR MEETING MY GOALS

DAILY GOAL TRACKER

(PLACE A STICKER OR CHECKMARK IF GOALS WERE ACHIEVED)

Mon	Tue	Wed	Thu

Fri	Sat	Sun

DAILY FOOD DIARY

DATE: ____________________ Ⓢ Ⓜ Ⓣ Ⓦ Ⓣ Ⓕ Ⓢ

TODAY'S GOALS *(IF ANY)*

GOAL MET?

BREAKFAST

LUNCH

DINNER

TOMORROW I LOOK FORWARD TO:

WATER / MILK INTAKE

TODAY I FELT...

DAILY FOOD DIARY

DATE: ____________________ Ⓢ Ⓜ Ⓣ Ⓦ Ⓣ Ⓕ Ⓢ

TODAY'S GOALS *(IF ANY)*

GOAL MET?

BREAKFAST

LUNCH

DINNER

TOMORROW I LOOK FORWARD TO:

WATER / MILK INTAKE

TODAY I FELT...

DAILY FOOD DIARY

DATE: ____________________ Ⓢ Ⓜ Ⓣ Ⓦ Ⓣ Ⓕ Ⓢ

TODAY'S GOALS *(IF ANY)*

GOAL MET?

BREAKFAST

LUNCH

DINNER

TOMORROW I LOOK FORWARD TO:

WATER / MILK INTAKE

TODAY I FELT...

DAILY FOOD DIARY

DATE: ____________________ (S) (M) (T) (W) (T) (F) (S)

TODAY'S GOALS *(IF ANY)*

GOAL MET?

BREAKFAST

LUNCH

DINNER

TOMORROW I LOOK FORWARD TO:

WATER / MILK INTAKE

TODAY I FELT...

DAILY FOOD DIARY

DATE: ______________________ Ⓢ Ⓜ Ⓣ Ⓦ Ⓣ Ⓕ Ⓢ

TODAY'S GOALS *(IF ANY)*

GOAL MET?

BREAKFAST

LUNCH

DINNER

TOMORROW I LOOK FORWARD TO:

WATER / MILK INTAKE

TODAY I FELT...

DAILY FOOD DIARY

DATE: ______________________ (S) (M) (T) (W) (T) (F) (S)

TODAY'S GOALS *(IF ANY)*

GOAL MET?

BREAKFAST

LUNCH

DINNER

TOMORROW I LOOK FORWARD TO:

WATER / MILK INTAKE

TODAY I FELT...

DAILY FOOD DIARY

DATE: ______________________ S M T W T F S

TODAY'S GOALS *(IF ANY)*

GOAL MET?

BREAKFAST

LUNCH

DINNER

TOMORROW I LOOK FORWARD TO:

WATER / MILK INTAKE

TODAY I FELT...

WEEK 2 REFLECTION

DATE: ____________________

THIS WEEK I FELT...

NEW FOODS I TRIED THIS WEEK:

-
-
-

FAVORITE FOODS

-
-
-
-

LEAST FAVORITE FOODS

-
-
-
-

NEXT WEEK I LOOK FORWARD TO:

WEEK 3

WEEK 3 FOOD GOALS

WEEK OF: ______________________

THIS WEEK'S GOALS

-
-
-

THIS WEEK'S REWARD FOR MEETING MY GOALS

DAILY GOAL TRACKER

(PLACE A STICKER OR CHECKMARK IF GOALS WERE ACHIEVED)

Mon Tue Wed Thu

Fri Sat Sun

DAILY FOOD DIARY

DATE: ____________________ Ⓢ Ⓜ Ⓣ Ⓦ Ⓣ Ⓕ Ⓢ

TODAY'S GOALS *(IF ANY)*

GOAL MET?

BREAKFAST

LUNCH

DINNER

TOMORROW I LOOK FORWARD TO:

WATER / MILK INTAKE

TODAY I FELT...

DAILY FOOD DIARY

DATE: ______________________ (S) (M) (T) (W) (T) (F) (S)

TODAY'S GOALS *(IF ANY)* GOAL MET?

BREAKFAST

LUNCH

DINNER

TOMORROW I LOOK FORWARD TO:

WATER / MILK INTAKE

TODAY I FELT...

DAILY FOOD DIARY

DATE: ____________________ S M T W T F S

TODAY'S GOALS *(IF ANY)*

GOAL MET?

BREAKFAST

LUNCH

DINNER

TOMORROW I LOOK FORWARD TO:

WATER / MILK INTAKE

TODAY I FELT...

DAILY FOOD DIARY

DATE: ____________________ Ⓢ Ⓜ Ⓣ Ⓦ Ⓣ Ⓕ Ⓢ

TODAY'S GOALS *(IF ANY)*

GOAL MET?

BREAKFAST

LUNCH

DINNER

TOMORROW I LOOK FORWARD TO:

WATER / MILK INTAKE

TODAY I FELT...

DAILY FOOD DIARY

DATE: ______________________ (S) (M) (T) (W) (T) (F) (S)

TODAY'S GOALS *(IF ANY)*

GOAL MET?

BREAKFAST

LUNCH

DINNER

TOMORROW I LOOK FORWARD TO:

WATER / MILK INTAKE

TODAY I FELT...

DAILY FOOD DIARY

DATE: ______________________ Ⓢ Ⓜ Ⓣ Ⓦ Ⓣ Ⓕ Ⓢ

TODAY'S GOALS *(IF ANY)*

GOAL MET?

BREAKFAST

LUNCH

DINNER

TOMORROW I LOOK FORWARD TO:

WATER / MILK INTAKE

TODAY I FELT...

DAILY FOOD DIARY

DATE: ______________________ Ⓢ Ⓜ Ⓣ Ⓦ Ⓣ Ⓕ Ⓢ

TODAY'S GOALS *(IF ANY)*

GOAL MET?

BREAKFAST

LUNCH

DINNER

TOMORROW I LOOK FORWARD TO:

WATER / MILK INTAKE

TODAY I FELT...

WEEK 3 REFLECTION

DATE: ____________________

THIS WEEK I FELT...

NEW FOODS I TRIED THIS WEEK:

FAVORITE FOODS

LEAST FAVORITE FOODS

NEXT WEEK I LOOK FORWARD TO:

WEEK 4

WEEK 4 FOOD GOALS

WEEK OF: ____________________

THIS WEEK'S GOALS

-
-
-

THIS WEEK'S REWARD FOR MEETING MY GOALS

DAILY GOAL TRACKER

(PLACE A STICKER OR CHECKMARK IF GOALS WERE ACHIEVED)

Mon	Tue	Wed	Thu

Fri	Sat	Sun

DAILY FOOD DIARY

DATE: ______________________ (S) (M) (T) (W) (T) (F) (S)

TODAY'S GOALS *(IF ANY)*

GOAL MET?

BREAKFAST

LUNCH

DINNER

TOMORROW I LOOK FORWARD TO:

WATER / MILK INTAKE

TODAY I FELT...

DAILY FOOD DIARY

DATE: ____________________ S M T W T F S

TODAY'S GOALS *(IF ANY)*

GOAL MET?

BREAKFAST

LUNCH

DINNER

TOMORROW I LOOK FORWARD TO:

WATER / MILK INTAKE

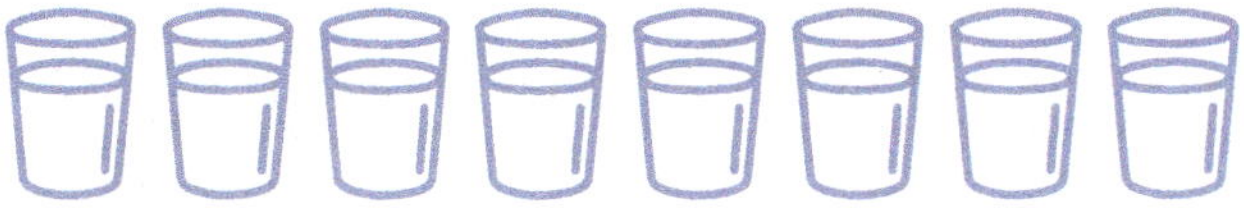

TODAY I FELT...

DAILY FOOD DIARY

DATE: ______________________ Ⓢ Ⓜ Ⓣ Ⓦ Ⓣ Ⓕ Ⓢ

TODAY'S GOALS *(IF ANY)*

GOAL MET?

BREAKFAST

LUNCH

DINNER

TOMORROW I LOOK FORWARD TO:

WATER / MILK INTAKE

TODAY I FELT...

DAILY FOOD DIARY

DATE: ____________________ (S) (M) (T) (W) (T) (F) (S)

TODAY'S GOALS *(IF ANY)*

GOAL MET?

-
-
-

BREAKFAST

-
-
-
-

LUNCH

-
-
-
-

DINNER

-
-
-
-

TOMORROW I LOOK FORWARD TO:

WATER / MILK INTAKE

TODAY I FELT...

DAILY FOOD DIARY

DATE: ______________________ (S) (M) (T) (W) (T) (F) (S)

TODAY'S GOALS *(IF ANY)* GOAL MET?

BREAKFAST

LUNCH

DINNER

TOMORROW I LOOK FORWARD TO:

WATER / MILK INTAKE

TODAY I FELT...

DAILY FOOD DIARY

DATE: ____________________ Ⓢ Ⓜ Ⓣ Ⓦ Ⓣ Ⓕ Ⓢ

TODAY'S GOALS *(IF ANY)*

GOAL MET?

BREAKFAST

LUNCH

DINNER

TOMORROW I LOOK FORWARD TO:

WATER / MILK INTAKE

TODAY I FELT...

DAILY FOOD DIARY

DATE: ______________________ (S) (M) (T) (W) (T) (F) (S)

TODAY'S GOALS *(IF ANY)*

GOAL MET?

BREAKFAST

LUNCH

DINNER

TOMORROW I LOOK FORWARD TO:

WATER / MILK INTAKE

TODAY I FELT...

WEEK 4 REFLECTION

DATE: ______________________

THIS WEEK I FELT...

NEW FOODS I TRIED THIS WEEK:

FAVORITE FOODS

LEAST FAVORITE FOODS

NEXT WEEK I LOOK FORWARD TO:

WEEK 5

WEEK 5 FOOD GOALS

WEEK OF: ____________________

THIS WEEK'S GOALS

-
-
-

THIS WEEK'S REWARD FOR MEETING MY GOALS

DAILY GOAL TRACKER

(PLACE A STICKER OR CHECKMARK IF GOALS WERE ACHIEVED)

Mon Tue Wed Thu

Fri Sat Sun

DAILY FOOD DIARY

DATE: ______________________ (S) (M) (T) (W) (T) (F) (S)

TODAY'S GOALS *(IF ANY)* GOAL MET?

BREAKFAST

LUNCH

DINNER

TOMORROW I LOOK FORWARD TO:

WATER / MILK INTAKE

TODAY I FELT...

DAILY FOOD DIARY

DATE: ______________________ Ⓢ Ⓜ Ⓣ Ⓦ Ⓣ Ⓕ Ⓢ

TODAY'S GOALS *(IF ANY)*

GOAL MET?

BREAKFAST

LUNCH

DINNER

TOMORROW I LOOK FORWARD TO:

WATER / MILK INTAKE

TODAY I FELT...

DAILY FOOD DIARY

DATE: ____________________ Ⓢ Ⓜ Ⓣ Ⓦ Ⓣ Ⓕ Ⓢ

TODAY'S GOALS *(IF ANY)*

GOAL MET?

BREAKFAST

LUNCH

DINNER

TOMORROW I LOOK FORWARD TO:

WATER / MILK INTAKE

TODAY I FELT...

DAILY FOOD DIARY

DATE: ______________________ (S) (M) (T) (W) (T) (F) (S)

TODAY'S GOALS *(IF ANY)* GOAL MET?

BREAKFAST

LUNCH

DINNER

TOMORROW I LOOK FORWARD TO:

WATER / MILK INTAKE

TODAY I FELT...

DAILY FOOD DIARY

DATE: ______________________ (S) (M) (T) (W) (T) (F) (S)

TODAY'S GOALS *(IF ANY)*

GOAL MET?

BREAKFAST

LUNCH

DINNER

TOMORROW I LOOK FORWARD TO:

WATER / MILK INTAKE

TODAY I FELT...

DAILY FOOD DIARY

DATE: ______________________ (S) (M) (T) (W) (T) (F) (S)

TODAY'S GOALS *(IF ANY)* GOAL MET?

BREAKFAST

LUNCH

DINNER

TOMORROW I LOOK FORWARD TO:

WATER / MILK INTAKE

TODAY I FELT...

DAILY FOOD DIARY

DATE: ____________________ (S) (M) (T) (W) (T) (F) (S)

TODAY'S GOALS *(IF ANY)* GOAL MET?

BREAKFAST

LUNCH

DINNER

TOMORROW I LOOK FORWARD TO:

WATER / MILK INTAKE

TODAY I FELT...

WEEK 5 REFLECTION

DATE: ______________________

THIS WEEK I FELT...

NEW FOODS I TRIED THIS WEEK:

-
-
-

FAVORITE FOODS

-
-
-
-

LEAST FAVORITE FOODS

-
-
-
-

NEXT WEEK I LOOK FORWARD TO:

WEEK 6

WEEK 6 FOOD GOALS

WEEK OF: ______________________

THIS WEEK'S GOALS

-
-
-

THIS WEEK'S REWARD FOR MEETING MY GOALS

DAILY GOAL TRACKER

(PLACE A STICKER OR CHECKMARK IF GOALS WERE ACHIEVED)

Mon Tue Wed Thu

Fri Sat Sun

DAILY FOOD DIARY

DATE: ______________________ (S) (M) (T) (W) (T) (F) (S)

TODAY'S GOALS *(IF ANY)*

GOAL MET?

BREAKFAST

LUNCH

DINNER

TOMORROW I LOOK FORWARD TO:

WATER / MILK INTAKE

TODAY I FELT...

DAILY FOOD DIARY

DATE: ______________________ (S) (M) (T) (W) (T) (F) (S)

TODAY'S GOALS *(IF ANY)*

GOAL MET?

BREAKFAST

LUNCH

DINNER

TOMORROW I LOOK FORWARD TO:

WATER / MILK INTAKE

TODAY I FELT...

DAILY FOOD DIARY

DATE: ____________________ S M T W T F S

TODAY'S GOALS *(IF ANY)*

GOAL MET?

BREAKFAST

LUNCH

DINNER

TOMORROW I LOOK FORWARD TO:

WATER / MILK INTAKE

TODAY I FELT...

DAILY FOOD DIARY

DATE: ______________________ (S) (M) (T) (W) (T) (F) (S)

TODAY'S GOALS *(IF ANY)*

GOAL MET?

BREAKFAST

LUNCH

DINNER

TOMORROW I LOOK FORWARD TO:

WATER / MILK INTAKE

TODAY I FELT...

DAILY FOOD DIARY

DATE: ______________________ S M T W T F S

TODAY'S GOALS *(IF ANY)* GOAL MET?

BREAKFAST

LUNCH

DINNER

TOMORROW I LOOK FORWARD TO:

WATER / MILK INTAKE

TODAY I FELT...

DAILY FOOD DIARY

DATE: ______________________ S M T W T F S

TODAY'S GOALS *(IF ANY)*

GOAL MET?

BREAKFAST

LUNCH

DINNER

TOMORROW I LOOK FORWARD TO:

WATER / MILK INTAKE

TODAY I FELT...

DAILY FOOD DIARY

DATE: ____________________ (S) (M) (T) (W) (T) (F) (S)

TODAY'S GOALS *(IF ANY)*

GOAL MET?

BREAKFAST

LUNCH

DINNER

TOMORROW I LOOK FORWARD TO:

WATER / MILK INTAKE

TODAY I FELT...

WEEK 6 REFLECTION

DATE: ______________________

THIS WEEK I FELT...

NEW FOODS I TRIED THIS WEEK:

-
-
-

FAVORITE FOODS

-
-
-
-

LEAST FAVORITE FOODS

-
-
-
-

NEXT WEEK I LOOK FORWARD TO:

WEEK 7

WEEK 7 FOOD GOALS

WEEK OF: ______________________

THIS WEEK'S GOALS

-
-
-

THIS WEEK'S REWARD FOR MEETING MY GOALS

DAILY GOAL TRACKER

(PLACE A STICKER OR CHECKMARK IF GOALS WERE ACHIEVED)

Mon Tue Wed Thu

Fri Sat Sun

DAILY FOOD DIARY

DATE: ____________________ Ⓢ Ⓜ Ⓣ Ⓦ Ⓣ Ⓕ Ⓢ

TODAY'S GOALS *(IF ANY)*

GOAL MET?

BREAKFAST

LUNCH

DINNER

TOMORROW I LOOK FORWARD TO:

WATER / MILK INTAKE

TODAY I FELT...

DAILY FOOD DIARY

DATE: ______________________ (S) (M) (T) (W) (T) (F) (S)

TODAY'S GOALS *(IF ANY)*

GOAL MET?

BREAKFAST

LUNCH

DINNER

TOMORROW I LOOK FORWARD TO:

WATER / MILK INTAKE

TODAY I FELT...

DAILY FOOD DIARY

DATE: ____________________ Ⓢ Ⓜ Ⓣ Ⓦ Ⓣ Ⓕ Ⓢ

TODAY'S GOALS *(IF ANY)*

GOAL MET?

BREAKFAST

LUNCH

DINNER

TOMORROW I LOOK FORWARD TO:

WATER / MILK INTAKE

TODAY I FELT...

DAILY FOOD DIARY

DATE: ____________________ Ⓢ Ⓜ Ⓣ Ⓦ Ⓣ Ⓕ Ⓢ

TODAY'S GOALS *(IF ANY)*

GOAL MET?

BREAKFAST

LUNCH

DINNER

TOMORROW I LOOK FORWARD TO:

WATER / MILK INTAKE

TODAY I FELT...

DAILY FOOD DIARY

DATE: ____________________ Ⓢ Ⓜ Ⓣ Ⓦ Ⓣ Ⓕ Ⓢ

TODAY'S GOALS *(IF ANY)*

GOAL MET?

BREAKFAST

LUNCH

DINNER

TOMORROW I LOOK FORWARD TO:

WATER / MILK INTAKE

TODAY I FELT...

DAILY FOOD DIARY

DATE: ______________________ S M T W T F S

TODAY'S GOALS *(IF ANY)*

GOAL MET?

BREAKFAST

LUNCH

DINNER

TOMORROW I LOOK FORWARD TO:

WATER / MILK INTAKE

TODAY I FELT...

DAILY FOOD DIARY

DATE: ____________________ Ⓢ Ⓜ Ⓣ Ⓦ Ⓣ Ⓕ Ⓢ

TODAY'S GOALS *(IF ANY)*

GOAL MET?

BREAKFAST

LUNCH

DINNER

TOMORROW I LOOK FORWARD TO:

WATER / MILK INTAKE

TODAY I FELT...

WEEK 7 REFLECTION

DATE: ______________________

THIS WEEK I FELT...

NEW FOODS I TRIED THIS WEEK:

FAVORITE FOODS

LEAST FAVORITE FOODS

NEXT WEEK I LOOK FORWARD TO:

WEEK 8

WEEK 8 FOOD GOALS

WEEK OF: ______________________

THIS WEEK'S GOALS

-
-
-

THIS WEEK'S REWARD FOR MEETING MY GOALS

DAILY GOAL TRACKER

(PLACE A STICKER OR CHECKMARK IF GOALS WERE ACHIEVED)

Mon

Tue

Wed

Thu

Fri

Sat

Sun

DAILY FOOD DIARY

DATE: ____________________

S M T W T F S

TODAY'S GOALS *(IF ANY)*

GOAL MET?

BREAKFAST

LUNCH

DINNER

TOMORROW I LOOK FORWARD TO:

WATER / MILK INTAKE

TODAY I FELT...

DAILY FOOD DIARY

DATE: ____________________ Ⓢ Ⓜ Ⓣ Ⓦ Ⓣ Ⓕ Ⓢ

TODAY'S GOALS *(IF ANY)* GOAL MET?

BREAKFAST

LUNCH

DINNER

TOMORROW I LOOK FORWARD TO:

WATER / MILK INTAKE

TODAY I FELT...

DAILY FOOD DIARY

DATE: ______________________ (S) (M) (T) (W) (T) (F) (S)

TODAY'S GOALS *(IF ANY)* GOAL MET?

BREAKFAST

LUNCH

DINNER

TOMORROW I LOOK FORWARD TO:

WATER / MILK INTAKE

TODAY I FELT...

DAILY FOOD DIARY

DATE: ______________________ (S) (M) (T) (W) (T) (F) (S)

TODAY'S GOALS *(IF ANY)*

GOAL MET?

BREAKFAST

LUNCH

DINNER

TOMORROW I LOOK FORWARD TO:

WATER / MILK INTAKE

TODAY I FELT...

DAILY FOOD DIARY

DATE: ____________________ (S) (M) (T) (W) (T) (F) (S)

TODAY'S GOALS *(IF ANY)*

GOAL MET?

BREAKFAST

LUNCH

DINNER

TOMORROW I LOOK FORWARD TO:

WATER / MILK INTAKE

TODAY I FELT...

DAILY FOOD DIARY

DATE: ______________________ S M T W T F S

TODAY'S GOALS *(IF ANY)*

GOAL MET?

BREAKFAST

LUNCH

DINNER

TOMORROW I LOOK FORWARD TO:

WATER / MILK INTAKE

TODAY I FELT...

DAILY FOOD DIARY

DATE: ____________________ Ⓢ Ⓜ Ⓣ Ⓦ Ⓣ Ⓕ Ⓢ

TODAY'S GOALS *(IF ANY)*

GOAL MET?

BREAKFAST

LUNCH

DINNER

TOMORROW I LOOK FORWARD TO:

WATER / MILK INTAKE

TODAY I FELT...

WEEK 8 REFLECTION

DATE: ____________________

THIS WEEK I FELT...

NEW FOODS I TRIED THIS WEEK:

-
-
-

FAVORITE FOODS

-
-
-
-

LEAST FAVORITE FOODS

-
-
-
-

NEXT WEEK I LOOK FORWARD TO:

Made in the USA
Monee, IL
02 November 2026

67379653R00046